The Bloating Solution

Practical steps to a flatter stomach and better health

Janet Bliss

Disclaimer

Please keep in mind that the content in this book is solely for educational purposes. The information offered here is said to be reliable and trustworthy. The author makes no implication or intends to offer any warranty of accuracy for particular individual cases.
Before beginning any diet or lifestyle habits, it is recommended that you contact a knowledgeable practitioner, such as your doctor. This book's material should not be utilized in place of expert counsel or professional guidance.
The author, publisher, and distributor expressly disclaim all liability, loss, damage, or danger incurred by persons who rely on the information in this book, whether directly or indirectly.
All intellectual property rights are retained. This book's information should not be replicated in any way, mechanically, electronically, photocopying, or by any other methods accessible

Table Of Contents

Chapter 1: "Emily's Journey to Digestive Freedom"

Emily was tired of feeling weighed down by constant bloating. For years, she battled discomfort after meals, struggling to find a solution. But one day, determined to take control of her digestive health, she embarked on a journey that would change her life.

As Emily sat across from me in my office, sharing her frustration and longing for relief, we discussed various approaches to tackle her bloating. Together, we explored the potential triggers and solutions, creating a personalized plan tailored to her needs.

With guidance, Emily made subtle yet impactful changes to her diet, incorporating probiotic-rich foods like yogurt and kefir while embracing fiber-packed options such as bananas and whole grains. She discovered the soothing effects of chamomile tea and the digestive aid found in ginger tea, integrating these herbal remedies into her daily routine.

Emily didn't stop there. Empowered by newfound knowledge, she explored yoga and Pilates, finding solace in poses that targeted her abdomen, aiding in the release of trapped gas. Her journey included a balance of exercise and hydration, discovering that a brisk walk after meals helped ease her digestion.

The transformation didn't happen overnight. It was a gradual process of learning, experimenting, and fine-tuning her approach. Emily found solace in the journey itself, embracing each step forward as a victory toward reclaiming her digestive comfort.
As weeks turned into months, Emily noticed remarkable changes. The discomfort that once shadowed her every meal began to fade. Her bloating reduced significantly, and she regained a sense of control over her digestive health.

Emily's success story is a testament to the power of personalized dietary adjustments, herbal remedies, and embracing a holistic approach to digestive wellness. Her journey serves as an inspiration, reminding us that with dedication, knowledge, and a willingness to explore, relief from bloating and digestive discomfort is within reach.

Chapter 2: Understanding Bloating

Bloating is a common and often uncomfortable sensation characterized by a feeling of fullness, tightness, or swelling in the abdomen. To truly address bloating, it's vital to delve into its intricate nature, encompassing its various forms, causes, and effects on daily life.

Bloating is not a one-size-fits-all condition. It manifests differently for each individual and can stem from multiple factors. Understanding the complexity involves recognizing the distinction between bloating and other digestive discomforts like gas or distention. Bloating often involves an excessive sensation of fullness or swelling that isn't necessarily relieved by burping or passing gas.

Bloating isn't merely a physical discomfort; it can significantly affect one's quality of life. This section addresses the pervasive impact of bloating on daily activities, social interactions, work performance, and emotional well-being. The psychological toll of chronic bloating, including its influence on body image and self-esteem, is explored to underscore its multifaceted consequences.

By comprehensively dissecting the intricacies of bloating, individuals gain a deeper insight into its nuanced nature. Recognizing the broad spectrum of causes and effects allows for a more holistic and effective approach toward finding personalized solutions for relief. Understanding that bloating is a multifactorial issue empowers individuals to navigate their journey towards a bloat-free existence with informed choices and tailored strategies.

Chapter 3: Types and Causes of Bloating

Types of Bloating:

1: Gas-related Bloating: This type of bloating occurs due to the accumulation of gas in the digestive system, leading to abdominal discomfort, fullness, and distention. It's often associated with excessive gas production or difficulty expelling gas.

2: Water Retention Bloating: Sometimes, bloating can be caused by water retention, leading to a feeling of swelling or puffiness in the abdomen. This can be influenced by factors such as hormonal fluctuations, high sodium intake, or certain medical conditions.

3: Food Sensitivity Bloating: Certain foods can trigger bloating in susceptible individuals. High-FODMAP foods (fermentable oligosaccharides, disaccharides, monosaccharides, and polyols), gluten, dairy, and artificial sweeteners are common culprits.

Causes of Bloating:

1: Digestive Issues: Conditions like irritable bowel syndrome (IBS), inflammatory bowel disease (IBD), celiac disease, lactose intolerance, or small intestinal bacterial overgrowth (SIBO) can cause bloating. These conditions disrupt normal digestive processes, leading to bloating as a symptom.

2: Gas Production: Eating certain foods high in carbohydrates, particularly those that are hard to digest, can result in increased gas production in the gut. This includes foods like beans, cabbage, onions, and carbonated drinks.

3: Swallowing Air: Habitual habits like eating too quickly, drinking through a straw, or chewing gum can lead to swallowing excess air, which accumulates in the digestive system, causing bloating.

4: Stress and Anxiety: Emotional stress can impact digestion by altering gut motility and triggering discomfort and bloating. The gut-brain connection plays a significant role in how stress affects digestive health.

5: Hormonal Changes: Women may experience bloating due to hormonal fluctuations during menstruation, pregnancy, or menopause, leading to water retention and abdominal discomfort.

Chapter 4: Dietary Culprits

Understanding the role of diet in bloating is paramount to finding effective solutions. This chapter meticulously explores the intricate relationship between what we eat and the onset of bloating, guiding readers to identify dietary triggers, achieve a balanced diet for digestive health, and comprehend the impact of hydration.

1: Identifying Trigger Foods

Unveiling the specific foods that trigger bloating is a crucial step in managing this discomfort. Detailed guidance is provided on recognizing and eliminating potential culprits such as high-FODMAP foods (fermentable oligosaccharides, disaccharides, monosaccharides, and polyols), gluten, dairy, cruciferous vegetables, and carbonated beverages. The chapter delves into how these foods can ferment in the gut, leading to gas production and bloating.

2: Balancing Your Diet for Digestive Health

This section offers comprehensive advice on crafting a diet conducive to digestive wellness. Strategies include incorporating fiber-rich foods gradually, opting for lean proteins, choosing whole grains, and embracing a variety of fruits and vegetables while considering individual tolerance levels. The concept of mindful eating to aid digestion and prevent overeating is emphasized, promoting an awareness of portion sizes and eating habits.

3: The Role of Water and Hydration
Water's crucial role in digestive health is elucidated, emphasizing the importance of adequate hydration. The chapter discusses how dehydration can exacerbate bloating and digestive discomfort, highlighting practical tips for staying properly hydrated throughout the day.

Chapter 5: Gut Health and Bloating

Delving into the intricate world of gut health provides a deeper understanding of its pivotal role in managing bloating. This chapter illuminates the nuances of the gut microbiome, strategies to enhance gut health, and the impact of probiotics and prebiotics in addressing bloating.

Gut Microbiome Explained:

Breakdown of the gut microbiome:
1. Diversity: The gut microbiome is incredibly diverse, comprising thousands of different species of bacteria alone. This diversity is essential for its proper functioning, as a wider range of bacterial species promotes a healthier gut environment.

2. Balance: A healthy gut microbiome is characterized by a delicate balance between beneficial and potentially harmful microorganisms. This balance is crucial for

supporting digestive processes, aiding in nutrient absorption, and protecting against harmful pathogens.

3. Functions: The gut microbiome is involved in various functions, such as breaking down dietary fiber that the human body can't digest on its own. This process produces short-chain fatty acids, which provide energy for the cells lining the colon and help maintain gut health.

4. Immune System Regulation: The gut microbiome plays a vital role in regulating the immune system. It interacts with the immune cells in the gut, influencing their development and activity, thereby impacting overall immune function.

5. Metabolism and Weight Regulation: Studies suggest that the gut microbiome may influence metabolism and weight regulation. Certain gut bacteria can affect how calories are extracted from food and stored, potentially impacting body weight.

6. Brain-Gut Axis: The gut microbiome communicates bidirectionally with the brain through what's known as the gut-brain axis. This connection influences brain function, mood, and behavior. Emerging research suggests that an imbalance in the gut microbiome may be linked to certain mental health conditions.

Factors like diet, lifestyle, medications (especially antibiotics), genetics, and environmental exposures can influence the composition and balance of the gut microbiome. Maintaining a diverse and balanced gut microbiome is key to supporting overall health, including digestive comfort and well-being. Strategies like consuming a varied diet rich in fiber, probiotics, and prebiotics, managing stress, regular exercise, and adequate sleep play crucial roles in nurturing a healthy gut microbiome.

Chapter 6: Strategies to Improve Gut Health

1. Dietary Adjustments: Incorporate a diverse range of fruits, vegetables, whole grains, and legumes into your diet. Focus on high-fiber foods, as they promote the growth of beneficial gut bacteria. Additionally, fermented foods like yogurt, kefir, kimchi, sauerkraut, and miso contain probiotics that support gut health.

2. Prebiotics and Probiotics: Prebiotics are types of fiber that feed the good bacteria in your gut. They are found in foods like garlic, onions, bananas, asparagus, and whole grains.

Probiotics, found in fermented foods and supplements, contain live beneficial bacteria that contribute to a healthy gut microbiome.

3. Reduce Intake of Artificial Additives: Limiting the consumption of artificial sweeteners, preservatives, and highly processed foods can positively impact gut health. These additives may disrupt the balance of gut bacteria, leading to digestive issues.
4. Manage Stress: Practices like meditation, deep breathing exercises, yoga, and mindfulness can help reduce stress levels. Stress management is crucial as it can impact gut health by altering gut motility and exacerbating digestive discomfort.

5. Adequate Hydration: Drinking enough water supports overall digestive function by aiding in the breakdown of food and the movement of waste through the digestive tract. Proper hydration helps maintain a healthy balance of gut bacteria.

6. Regular Exercise: Physical activity not only benefits overall health but also contributes to a healthy gut. Exercise promotes gut motility and can positively impact the diversity of gut microbes.

7. Adequate Sleep: Prioritize quality sleep, as insufficient or disrupted sleep patterns can negatively impact gut health. Establishing a consistent sleep routine supports the body's natural digestive processes.

8. Limit Antibiotic Use When Possible: Antibiotics can disrupt the balance of gut bacteria. When prescribed antibiotics, discuss with your healthcare provider about strategies to protect and restore gut health during and after the treatment.

Chapter 7: Holistic Remedies

Exploring holistic approaches to alleviate bloating encompasses a spectrum of natural remedies and practices that can effectively aid in reducing discomfort. This chapter delves into various holistic techniques, including herbal remedies, breathing exercises, and mindfulness practices, offering readers a comprehensive toolkit for managing bloating.

Herbal Teas and Natural Remedies

Herbal teas and natural remedies are often used to alleviate bloating and aid in digestive comfort. Here's a list of some commonly used herbal teas and natural remedies along with their potential benefits for reducing bloating:

1. Peppermint Tea: Peppermint contains menthol, which has anti-spasmodic properties that can help relax the muscles in the digestive tract. This relaxation may ease bloating and reduce discomfort by allowing trapped gas to pass more easily.
2. Chamomile Tea: Chamomile possesses anti-inflammatory properties and can help relax muscles in the digestive tract. It may soothe an upset stomach, reduce gas, and ease bloating.

3. Ginger Tea: Ginger has been traditionally used to aid digestion and alleviate gastrointestinal discomfort. It can help reduce inflammation in the gut, improve digestion, and ease bloating by promoting the movement of food through the digestive system.

4. Fennel Tea: Fennel seeds contain compounds that can relax the muscles in the gastrointestinal tract, reducing bloating and aiding digestion. They can help alleviate gas and bloating by supporting the expulsion of gas from the digestive system.

5. Dandelion Tea: Dandelion root tea is believed to have diuretic properties, promoting increased urination and potentially reducing water retention that contributes to bloating. It may also support liver function and aid digestion.

6. Lemon Water: Drinking warm lemon water can stimulate the digestive system and help flush out toxins. It may promote healthy digestion and reduce bloating by encouraging the release of digestive enzymes.

7. Activated Charcoal: Activated charcoal is thought to absorb excess gas in the digestive system, potentially reducing bloating. It binds to gas-producing compounds, aiding in their removal from the body.

8. Digestive Enzymes: Natural digestive enzyme supplements contain enzymes like amylase, protease, and lipase, which aid in breaking down carbohydrates, proteins, and fats. Taking these supplements with meals can support digestion and reduce bloating by enhancing nutrient absorption.

These herbal teas and natural remedies are commonly used to alleviate bloating and digestive discomfort. However, individual responses can vary, and it's essential to consult with a healthcare professional before incorporating new herbal remedies or supplements, especially if you have underlying health conditions, are pregnant, or are taking medications. Additionally, while these remedies may provide relief for occasional bloating, persistent or severe bloating should be evaluated by a healthcare provider to rule out underlying conditions.

Chapter 8: Exercises for bloating

Here's a list of exercises that can potentially help reduce bloating and explanations for how they may provide relief:

1. Walking: A simple and accessible exercise, walking stimulates digestion by promoting movement in the abdomen. It aids in the natural contractions of the intestines, facilitating the

passage of food and reducing the likelihood of bloating due to slowed digestion.

2. Yoga: Certain yoga poses can target the abdominal area, aiding in the release of trapped gas and promoting relaxation in the digestive system. Poses like Wind-Relieving Pose (Pavanamuktasana), Cat-Cow Pose (Marjaryasana-Bitilasana), and Seated Twist (Ardha Matsyendrasana) can help relieve bloating by stimulating digestion and encouraging gas release.

3. Pilates: Pilates exercises focus on core strength and stability. These movements engage the abdominal muscles, which can aid in improving digestion by promoting better muscle function in the abdomen and reducing abdominal discomfort.

4. Cycling: Cycling, whether outdoors or on a stationary bike, involves rhythmic movements that can stimulate the abdominal area. The pedaling motion engages the core muscles and

may aid in relieving gas and reducing bloating by promoting intestinal movement.

5. Aerobic Exercises: Cardiovascular exercises like jogging, running, or dancing can increase heart rate and improve overall circulation. Enhanced blood flow to the digestive organs may help support efficient digestion and reduce the likelihood of bloating.

6. Breathing Exercises: Diaphragmatic breathing or deep belly breathing exercises can help relax the abdominal muscles, ease tension, and improve overall digestion. By reducing stress and promoting relaxation, these techniques may indirectly help alleviate bloating associated with stress-induced digestive issues.

It's important to note that while these exercises may help alleviate bloating for some individuals, individual responses can vary. The effectiveness of exercise in reducing bloating also depends on the underlying causes of bloating in each person.

Consulting with a healthcare professional before starting any new exercise regimen is advisable, especially if you have existing health conditions or concerns related to bloating. Incorporating a variety of exercises into your routine and finding what works best for your body can contribute to better digestive health and reduced bloating over time.

Exercise offers various benefits that can help alleviate bloating and improve overall digestive health. Here are the key ways exercise can contribute to reducing bloating:

1. Promotes Gut Motility: Regular physical activity, such as walking, jogging, or yoga, can stimulate the muscles in the abdomen and promote gut motility. This movement assists in the smooth passage of food through the digestive tract, reducing the likelihood of bloating due to slowed digestion.

2. Reduces Constipation: Exercise helps regulate bowel movements by enhancing muscle contractions in the intestines. By preventing

constipation, exercise minimizes the buildup of waste in the colon, decreasing the chances of bloating and discomfort.

3. Aids Gas Release: Certain exercises, such as yoga poses targeting the abdomen, can help release trapped gas from the digestive system. Twisting and stretching movements in yoga can stimulate the abdominal organs, facilitating the release of excess gas that may cause bloating.

4. Manages Stress: Stress can contribute to digestive discomfort, including bloating. Exercise is a powerful stress-reliever, as it prompts the release of endorphins, which are natural mood elevators. Reduced stress levels can indirectly alleviate bloating triggered by stress-related digestive disturbances.

5. Improves Overall Digestive Health: Regular physical activity supports overall digestive health by maintaining a healthy weight, enhancing metabolism, and promoting a

balanced gut microbiome. A healthy digestive system is less prone to bloating and discomfort.

6. Enhances Circulation: Exercise improves blood flow and circulation throughout the body, including the digestive organs. Improved circulation aids in the efficient functioning of the digestive system, potentially reducing bloating by optimizing nutrient absorption and waste elimination.

By incorporating regular exercise into your routine, you can positively impact digestive processes, reduce stress, and enhance overall well-being. Aim for a combination of cardiovascular exercises, strength training, and flexibility exercises to support digestive health and alleviate bloating.

Chapter 9: Mindfulness and Bloating Connection

1. Stress Reduction: Mindfulness practices, such as meditation, deep breathing exercises, and guided imagery, help reduce stress levels. High-stress levels can negatively impact digestion,

triggering bloating and other gastrointestinal discomforts. By managing stress through mindfulness, individuals may experience reduced bloating as a result.

2. Improved Digestive Awareness: Mindfulness encourages individuals to pay attention to bodily sensations, including those related to digestion. By becoming more aware of how different foods and emotions affect their digestive system, individuals can identify triggers that may lead to bloating.

3. Mindful Eating: Practicing mindfulness during meals involves paying attention to the sensory experiences of eating—taste, texture, smell—and being aware of hunger cues and fullness. Mindful eating can lead to slower eating, improved chewing, and better digestion, reducing the likelihood of bloating caused by overeating or poor eating habits.

4. Reduced Tension in the Gut: Mindfulness practices often include relaxation techniques

that can reduce tension in the gastrointestinal tract. Relaxing the gut muscles can promote smoother digestion and decrease the likelihood of bloating or discomfort.

5. Mind-Body Connection: Mindfulness practices strengthen the mind-body connection. This connection influences various bodily functions, including digestion. By fostering a harmonious relationship between the mind and body, individuals may experience fewer instances of stress-induced bloating.

Chapter 10: Foods to avoid to stop and reduce bloating:

1. High-FODMAP Foods: Fermentable oligosaccharides, disaccharides, monosaccharides, and polyols are certain types of carbohydrates that can be poorly absorbed in the gut. Examples include:
   - Onions and Garlic: These contain fructans, a type of oligosaccharide that

some people find difficult to digest, leading to bloating.

- Wheat and Rye: High in fructans and can cause bloating in individuals sensitive to these carbohydrates.

2. Cruciferous Vegetables: Vegetables like broccoli, cauliflower, cabbage, and Brussels sprouts are high in fiber and raffinose, which can lead to gas production in the gut, causing bloating for some people.

3. Legumes: Beans, lentils, and peas contain carbohydrates that are not fully broken during digestion, leading to gas production and bloating in susceptible individuals.

4. Dairy Products: Lactose, the sugar found in dairy products, can cause bloating in individuals with lactose intolerance. This condition involves an inability to fully digest lactose due to a deficiency in the enzyme lactase.

5. Carbonated Beverages: The fizz in carbonated drinks contain gas (carbon dioxide), which can be trapped in the digestive system, leading to bloating and discomfort.

6. Artificial Sweeteners: Sugar alcohols like sorbitol, found in many sugar-free gums and candies, can cause bloating and gastrointestinal discomfort as they are poorly absorbed in the gut.

7. High-Fat Foods: Fatty foods can slow down digestion, leading to a feeling of fullness and bloating. Fried foods, rich sauces, and fatty meats might contribute to this discomfort.

8. Some Fruits: Apples, pears, and stone fruits like peaches and plums contain fructose, which can cause bloating in individuals with fructose malabsorption.

9. Salty Foods: Excessive sodium intake can lead to water retention, causing a feeling of bloating or puffiness. Processed and canned foods, salty snacks, and high-sodium condiments contribute to increased water retention.

10. Sugary Foods and Beverages: High-sugar foods and drinks can ferment in the gut, leading to gas production and bloating. Sugary treats, sweetened beverages, and high-fructose corn syrup can contribute to discomfort in some individuals.

11. Processed Foods: Many processed foods contain additives, preservatives, and artificial ingredients that some people find difficult to digest. These additives may disrupt the balance of gut bacteria, potentially leading to bloating and digestive discomfort.

12. Alcohol: Alcohol can irritate the gastrointestinal tract and affect gut motility,

leading to bloating, gas, and discomfort for some individuals. It can also cause dehydration, exacerbating bloating in some cases.

13.   Spicy Foods: Some spicy dishes can irritate the digestive tract, causing bloating, gas, or abdominal discomfort in susceptible individuals. They may also stimulate the production of stomach acid, contributing to digestive discomfort.

14.   High-Carb Foods: While carbohydrates are an essential part of a balanced diet, excessive consumption of refined carbohydrates like white bread, pastries, and sugary cereals can lead to rapid digestion and gas production, potentially causing bloating.

15.   Caffeinated Beverages: Coffee, tea, and energy drinks containing caffeine can act as diuretics, leading to increased urination and potential dehydration.

16.   Caffeine can also stimulate the digestive system, causing bloating and discomfort in some individuals.

17.   Chewing Gum: Chewing gum leads to swallowing air, which can accumulate in the digestive tract and cause bloating and gas. Additionally, sugar alcohols in sugar-free gums may contribute to bloating in sensitive individuals.

Chapter 11: Foods that helps during bloating and what to add into routine

Here's a list of foods to incorporate into your diet and dietary additions that may help alleviate bloating, along with explanations for their potential benefits in reducing bloating:

- Probiotic-Rich Foods: Foods containing probiotics introduce beneficial bacteria to the gut, promoting a healthy balance of gut flora. Examples include:
  - Yogurt: Contains live cultures of beneficial bacteria that support gut health and aid digestion, potentially reducing bloating.
  - Kefir: A fermented dairy product rich in probiotics that can contribute to a healthy gut microbiome and help alleviate bloating.

- Fiber-Rich Foods: High-fiber foods aid digestion and promote regular bowel movements, reducing constipation and bloating. eg:
  - Whole Grains: Brown rice, quinoa, oats, and whole wheat contain soluble fiber that helps soften stool and ease digestion.
  - Fruits and Vegetables: Berries, apples, bananas, spinach, kale, and carrots are high-fiber options that aid in digestion and prevent bloating by supporting regular bowel movements.

- Herbal Teas: Certain herbal teas have properties that aid digestion and reduce bloating:
    - Peppermint Tea: Contains menthol, which relaxes the muscles of the digestive tract, potentially reducing bloating and gas.
    - Ginger Tea: Known for its anti-inflammatory properties, ginger can soothe the digestive system and alleviate bloating by aiding digestion.

- Lean Proteins: Incorporate lean protein sources into your diet to support muscle function and aid in digestion:
    - Chicken, Turkey, Fish: These lean protein sources are easier to digest compared to fatty meats, potentially reducing the likelihood of bloating.
- Herbs and Spices: Certain herbs and spices can aid digestion and reduce bloating:
    - Turmeric: Contains curcumin, which has anti-inflammatory properties that may help soothe the digestive system and alleviate bloating.

o Cumin, Coriander, and Fennel Seeds: These seeds contain compounds that aid digestion, reduce gas, and alleviate bloating by promoting gas expulsion from the digestive tract.

- Hydration: Drinking plenty of water throughout the day helps maintain proper hydration, softens stool, and aids in regular bowel movements, reducing the chances of bloating.

- Herbal Remedies:
  o Chamomile: Chamomile tea has anti-inflammatory properties that may soothe the digestive tract, reducing bloating and discomfort.
  o Dandelion Tea: Dandelion root tea acts as a mild diuretic, potentially reducing water retention and bloating.

- Low-FODMAP Foods: For individuals sensitive to certain carbohydrates, a low-FODMAP diet may help reduce bloating. Low-FODMAP options include:

o Bananas: Ripe bananas are low in fermentable sugars and can be easier on the digestive system.

o Potatoes: Both white and sweet potatoes are low-FODMAP options that can be less likely to cause bloating in some individuals.

- Healthy Fats: Incorporating healthy fats into your diet can aid in digestion and potentially reduce bloating:

  o Avocado: Contains healthy fats and fiber that can support digestion and reduce bloating.

  o Nuts and Seeds: Almonds, walnuts, and chia seeds are rich in fiber and healthy fats, aiding in digestion and reducing bloating.

- Fermented Foods: Apart from yogurt and kefir, other fermented foods can support gut health:

  o Kimchi: A traditional Korean fermented vegetable dish rich in probiotics that can help balance gut bacteria and aid digestion.

  o Sauerkraut: Fermented cabbage that contains probiotics beneficial for gut health and reducing bloating.

- Digestive Enzymes: Enzyme supplements may aid digestion and reduce bloating by supporting the breakdown of food:
    o Papaya: Contains the enzyme papain, aiding in protein digestion and potentially reducing bloating.
- Apple Cider Vinegar: Some individuals find that consuming diluted apple cider vinegar before meals can support digestion and reduce bloating by promoting stomach acid production and aiding digestion.

Remember, individual responses to foods vary, and it's essential to pay attention to your body's reactions. Gradually incorporating these foods and dietary additions into your routine while maintaining a balanced diet can contribute to improved digestive comfort and reduced bloating. If you have specific dietary concerns or health conditions, it's advisable to consult with a healthcare professional or registered dietitian for personalized guidance.

Chapter 12: Bloating Myths Debunked

This chapter meticulously addresses prevalent misconceptions surrounding bloating, dissecting common myths, and offering evidence-based insights to distinguish between popular beliefs and scientific facts. Readers will gain a comprehensive understanding of various misconceptions and the truth behind them, empowering them to make informed decisions regarding bloating management.

Common Misconceptions

The chapter begins by outlining widespread misconceptions about bloating. It systematically dismantles myths, such as "bloating is always related to overeating," "all bloating is due to gas," or "bloating is a normal part of aging." By debunking these myths, readers are encouraged to challenge preconceived notions and recognize the multifaceted nature of bloating.

Popular Remedies vs. Scientific Facts

This section meticulously dissects commonly touted remedies or practices for managing bloating. It scrutinizes claims about miracle foods, restrictive diets, or trendy treatments that lack scientific evidence. Instead, readers are provided with evidence-based approaches and validated strategies supported by scientific research to effectively address bloating.

Navigating through Misinformation

Armed with critical thinking skills, readers learn how to discern credible sources of information from misleading content. This section equips individuals with tools to evaluate information about bloating found in media, advertisements, and online platforms, enabling them to make informed choices and avoid falling prey to misinformation.

By exposing and debunking prevalent myths, scrutinizing popular remedies, and empowering readers to navigate through the abundance of information available, this chapter serves as a reliable guide. It equips individuals with the knowledge and skills necessary to separate fact from fiction in their quest to manage bloating effectively and make informed decisions about their digestive health.

Chapter 13: Everyday Strategies for Bloating

This chapter delves into practical, everyday strategies designed to offer immediate relief and long-term management of bloating. Readers will explore quick fixes, proactive planning for social situations, and effective approaches to manage bloating during travel, providing a comprehensive toolkit for navigating various scenarios.

Quick Fixes and Immediate Relief
Readers are introduced to a range of quick-fix strategies to alleviate bloating when it strikes unexpectedly. These include gentle exercises like walking, specific yoga poses, abdominal massages, or acupressure techniques targeting key areas to promote gas release and ease discomfort.

Planning Ahead for Social Situations
Guidance is provided on navigating social situations where dietary triggers may be prevalent, such as parties, gatherings, or dining out. Readers learn proactive strategies, including menu scrutiny, communication techniques with hosts or restaurants, and alternative food choices, enabling them to enjoy social occasions without exacerbating bloating.

Traveling and Managing Bloating

Insights on managing bloating during travel, a common challenge due to changes in routine, diet, and stress levels, are meticulously outlined. Readers gain practical tips on staying hydrated, choosing travel-friendly foods, incorporating movement during transit, and adjusting to different time zones, allowing for a more comfortable travel experience.

By equipping readers with practical strategies for immediate relief, social scenarios, and travel situations, this chapter empowers individuals to navigate diverse circumstances while effectively managing bloating. Whether seeking quick relief or planning ahead for specific situations, readers gain a comprehensive set of tools to minimize discomfort and maintain digestive comfort in various everyday scenarios.

9 798872 873150